THE NEWLY DIAGNOSED GUIDE TO HASHIMOTO'S DIET

Nourishing recipes and healing process to Hashimoto's thyroiditis.

Kerry O. Smith

COPYRIGHT

TABLE OF CONTENTS

THE NEWLY DIAGNOSED GUIDE TO HASHIMOTO'S DIET 1

COPYRIGHT 2

INTRODUCTION 10

CHAPTER 1 14

Understanding Hashimoto's thyroiditis 14

Importance of diet in managing Hashimoto's 19

Overview of the 21-day elimination diet 23

Benefits of the 21-Day Elimination Diet: 26

Life after the elimination diet 28

CHAPTER 2: BREAKFAST 33

1. Mango Turmeric Lassi.................... 33

2. Tahini Squash Porridge 34

3. Veggie Scramble 36

4. Bright Green Detox Smoothie 37

5. Red Velvet Smoothie 38

6. Grain-Free Granola 40

7. Breakfast Sausage and Cauli-Hash .. 42

8. Banana-Walnut Almond Flour Muffins 43

9. Spinach and Herb Frittata 45

10. Raspberry Cinnamon Yogurt Bowl 47

11. Apple-Carrot Breakfast Muffins .. 48

12. Fruit and Coconut Yogurt Parfait . 50

CHAPTER 3: SNACKS AND TREATS .. 52

1. Homemade Cherry Gummies 52

2. Strawberry Fruit Tart 53

3. Slow Cooker Poached Pears............ 55

4. Spiced Walnuts 56

5. Avocado Deviled Eggs 58

6. Crispy, Crunchy Carrot Fries.......... 59

7. Kale Chips 61

8. Guacamole with Jicama................... 63

9. Zucchini Rounds with Tapenade 64

10. Refrigerator Dill Pickles............... 65

11. Plantain Chips................................ 67

12. Cherry Tiger-nut Flour Leather 68

CHAPTER 4: EASY VEGETABLES AND SIDES.. 70

1. Cold Asian Zoodle Salad 70

2. Baked Herbed Zucchini Boats........ 72

3. Creamy Pineapple Coleslaw............ 73

4. Stuffed Zucchini 75

5. Veggie "Rice" Bowl 77

6. Spaghetti Squash Marinara 78

7. Huevos Rancheros 81

8. Sweet Potato Curry 83

9. Balsamic Marinated Fennel Salad ... 85

10. Quick Pickled Red Onions 86

CHAPTER 5: MAIN SEAFOODS 89

1. Mahi-Mahi with Mango Agrodolce. 89

2. Pan-Roasted Halibut 91

3. Mexican Cod Fish Tacos 92

4. Ginger-Spiced Tuna Salad Wraps.... 94

5. Shrimp Curry 96

6. Shrimp Cauliflower Fried Rice 98

7. White Fish Red Curry 100

8. Poached Cod with Summer Vegetables and Quinoa 102

9. Spicy Shrimp, Okra, and Tomato Stew 104

10. Crab and Asparagus Casserole ... 106

CHAPTER 6: POULTRY AND MEAT .. 108

1. Nutty Chicken Lettuce Wraps 108

2. Lamb Shepherd's Pie 110

3. Creamy Beef Casserole 112

4. Turkey Piccata with Lemon Zucchini 113

5. Slow Cooker Sloppy Joe Bowls 115

6. Steak Fajitas with Onions and Peppers 117

7. Cucumber Salad..............................119

8. Meatloaf Meatballs Lettuce Wraps with Dipping Sauce 121

9. Unstuffed Cabbage Rolls................ 123

10. Cinnamon Lamb Skillet 125

11. Mediterranean Chicken Pizzas ... 126

12. One-Pot Zuppa Toscana 128

CHAPTER 7: DESSERTS 131

1. Vanilla-Chamomile Poached Plums 131

2. Apple-Pear Sauce 132

3. Cranberry-Orange Compote 134

4. Avocado-Chocolate Frozen Peaches and Cream Bars 135

5. Cool Mint and Honeydew Slushy . 137

6. Chocolate-Covered Blueberry-Coconut Bars 138

7. Orange Poached Pears with Nutmeg 140

CHAPTER 8: KITCHEN STAPLES 142

1. Coconut Cream 142

2. Italian Sausage 143

3. Hard-Boiled Eggs 145

4. Roasted Garlic 146

5. Slow Cooker Caramelized Onions 148

6. Homemade Mayonnaise 149

CONCLUSION 152

INTRODUCTION

Hello, I'm Joan, and at the age of 18, I found myself grappling with the challenges of thyroiditis. It wasn't just a health hurdle; it became a financial strain for my parents.

The medical bills piled up, and the journey was tough. Fast forward to today, and I can share a story of transformation, resilience, and hope, thanks to the aid of my tailored diet and an incredible book.

Back then, thyroiditis cast a shadow over my life. It was a time of uncertainty and discomfort, not just for me but for my family. The strain on my parents, both emotionally and financially, was palpable. Medical bills seemed to cascade like an insurmountable mountain, and I felt the weight of their sacrifices.

However, five years down the road, the narrative has shifted. My journey took a positive turn when I stumbled upon a book that became my guide and confidant.

Its pages unfolded a roadmap to navigate the intricate dance between thyroiditis and nutrition. With the help of my personalized diet, I discovered a newfound strength, both physically and emotionally.

This book became a beacon of light, not only outlining the 21-Day Elimination Diet but also weaving practical tips, flavorful recipes, and heartfelt advice into my story.

Each chapter resonated with my experiences, turning what could have been a mundane dietary plan into a culinary adventure.

As I delved into the cookbook section, I found joy in preparing meals that not only supported my health but also satisfied my taste buds. Week after week, the pages of my medical diary documented a metamorphosis – a shift from vulnerability to empowerment.

The reintroduction of previously eliminated foods in Week 3 felt like a celebration of progress. Dining out became a manageable experience, and social gatherings turned into opportunities to showcase the delicious possibilities of a Hashimoto's-friendly diet.

Today, I stand at the intersection of gratitude and resilience. The financial burden has eased, my health has improved, and I've learned to embrace a lifestyle that nurtures both my body and spirit.

This book has been a true companion in my journey, turning what seemed like a daunting diagnosis at 18 into a story of triumph at 23.

Dear reader, I hope that my journey inspires you. Life with thyroiditis can be challenging, but with the right guidance and a personalized diet, it can also be a journey of growth, healing, and unexpected joy.

CHAPTER 1

Understanding Hashimoto's thyroiditis

Hashimoto's thyroiditis is a condition where the immune system, our body's defense mechanism, mistakenly identifies the thyroid gland as a threat and launches an attack against it.

The thyroid, a small butterfly-shaped gland located in the neck, plays a crucial role in regulating various bodily functions by producing hormones.

These hormones, namely thyroxine (T4) and triiodothyronine (T3), influence metabolism, energy levels, and the functioning of organs.

In Hashimoto's, the immune system produces antibodies that target the thyroid, leading to inflammation and potential damage.

Over time, this chronic inflammation can impair the thyroid's ability to produce hormones efficiently, resulting in a condition known as hypothyroidism.

It is essential to note that not everyone with Hashimoto's thyroiditis will develop hypothyroidism, and the progression of the disease varies from person to person.

Recognizing the silent character of Hashimoto's is essential to comprehending the condition. In the early stages, people frequently don't detect any symptoms. It is a cunning attacker that subtly affects thyroid function without causing obvious symptoms.

Symptoms include weariness, weight gain, sensitivity to cold, dry skin, and muscle weakness may appear as the condition worsens.

Diagnosis typically involves blood tests to measure thyroid hormone levels and the presence of specific antibodies. Anti-thyroid peroxidase (TPO) antibodies and anti-thyroglobulin antibodies are commonly assessed to confirm the autoimmune nature of Hashimoto's.

Let's now examine the significance of this and possible solutions. Comprehending the autoimmune component is essential since it influences the therapeutic strategy.

Effective management techniques for autoimmune disorders try to reduce symptoms and maintain thyroid function, even though traditional medication may not be able to cure them.

One cornerstone of managing Hashimoto's is adopting a personalized and supportive lifestyle, starting with diet. Many individuals with Hashimoto's find relief by following a gluten-free diet. Gluten, a protein found in wheat and related grains, has been linked to autoimmune thyroid conditions.

Additionally, an anti-inflammatory diet rich in nutrient-dense foods, such as fruits, vegetables, and lean proteins, can be beneficial.

The concept of a 21-day elimination diet often comes into play, where certain foods are temporarily removed to identify potential triggers and sensitivities. This can serve as a reset for the immune system and digestive health.

Beyond dietary considerations, stress management plays a pivotal role. Chronic stress can exacerbate autoimmune conditions, including Hashimoto's. Incorporating relaxation techniques, regular exercise, and sufficient sleep can contribute to overall well-being.

In some cases, medication may be prescribed to supplement thyroid hormone levels and manage hypothyroidism. It's important to work closely with healthcare providers to find the right balance and dosage.

Comprehending the autoimmune nature of Hashimoto's thyroiditis, identifying possible symptoms, and adopting a comprehensive care strategy are essential to its knowledge. People can manage their stress, work with medical providers, and address dietary issues to help them achieve optimal well-being while navigating this condition with resilience.

Importance of diet in managing Hashimoto's

The role of diet in managing Hashimoto's thyroiditis is paramount, as it can significantly impact the symptoms and progression of this autoimmune condition.

In simpler terms, what you eat plays a crucial role in supporting your body's ability to navigate the challenges posed by Hashimoto's.

Hashimoto's involves the immune system mistakenly attacking the thyroid gland, leading to inflammation and potential damage. A well-thought-out diet can serve as a powerful tool to mitigate inflammation, optimize thyroid function, and enhance overall well-being.

Inflammation Control: Hashimoto's thyroiditis is characterized by chronic thyroid gland inflammation caused by an autoimmune reaction. An anti-inflammatory diet reduces inflammation, relieving thyroid strain and maybe decreasing disease progression.

Supporting Thyroid Function: Certain nutrients are vital for optimal thyroid function. A well-balanced diet, rich in essential vitamins and minerals like selenium, iodine, and zinc, ensures that the thyroid has the necessary building blocks to produce hormones effectively.

Balancing Immune Response: Diet can influence the immune system's behavior. By avoiding potential triggers and incorporating immune-supportive foods, individuals with

Hashimoto's may help regulate the immune response, reducing the severity of attacks on the thyroid.

Minimizing Symptoms: Hashimoto often presents with symptoms such as fatigue, weight gain, and mood disturbances. A diet tailored to individual needs can address nutritional deficiencies and contribute to overall well-being, potentially alleviating some of these symptoms.

Gluten Sensitivity: Many individuals with Hashimoto's experience sensitivity to gluten, a protein found in wheat and related grains. Going gluten-free may help reduce inflammation and improve symptoms for those with gluten sensitivity.

Blood Sugar Regulation: Maintaining stable blood sugar levels is essential for individuals with Hashimoto's. A diet focused on complex carbohydrates, fiber, and balanced meals can help regulate blood sugar, preventing energy crashes and supporting hormonal balance.

Gut Health: The health of the gut is closely linked to autoimmune conditions. An elimination diet and the inclusion of probiotic-rich foods can support a healthy gut microbiome, potentially reducing the autoimmune response seen in Hashimoto's.

Individualized Approach: Each person with Hashimoto's may respond differently to specific foods. Adopting an individualized approach, such as the 21-day elimination diet, allows individuals to identify and avoid foods that may trigger or worsen symptoms.

Preventing Nutrient Deficiencies: Hashimoto's can lead to nutrient deficiencies due to impaired absorption. A nutrient-dense diet helps prevent deficiencies and ensures the body has the resources it needs for optimal functioning.

Overview of the 21-day elimination diet

Hashimoto's thyroiditis is a condition characterized by an autoimmune response impacting the thyroid gland. Symptoms of Hashimoto's disease include fatigue, weight gain, and mood swings. The 21-day elimination diet is a method for identifying and eliminating potential triggers that may aggravate Hashimoto's symptoms.

Key Steps in the 21-Day Elimination Diet:

Remove Common Triggers: The first step is to eliminate certain foods known to contribute to inflammation and autoimmune reactions. These commonly include gluten, dairy, soy, and refined sugars.

Focus on Whole Foods: During the 21 days, emphasize whole, nutrient-dense foods like fruits, vegetables, lean proteins, and healthy fats. This aids in delivering necessary nutrients and promotes overall well-being.

Track Symptoms: Keep a journal to record changes in symptoms throughout the diet. This can help identify patterns and pinpoint specific foods that may be problematic.

Reintroduction Phase: After the elimination period, slowly reintroduce one eliminated food group at a time, allowing a few days between each reintroduction. Monitor for any adverse reactions or symptom flare-ups.

Personalized Approach: Every individual's response to foods can vary, so the 21-day elimination diet is a tool to identify a personalized and sustainable eating plan that supports optimal health for those with Hashimoto's.

Why the 21-Day Duration?

The 21-day timeframe is chosen as it aligns with the typical timeframe for the body to show noticeable reactions to dietary changes. It's a long enough period to allow the immune system to settle and for potential trigger foods to be cleared from the system.

Benefits of the 21-Day Elimination Diet:

Identifying Triggers: Pinpointing specific foods that may exacerbate Hashimoto's symptoms allows for a targeted and personalized approach to managing the condition.

Reducing Inflammation: By eliminating potentially inflammatory foods, the diet aims to reduce overall inflammation in the body, which is beneficial for autoimmune conditions like Hashimoto's.

Improved Well-Being: Many individuals report feeling better, with reduced fatigue and improved mood, after completing the 21-day elimination diet.

Important Considerations:

Consult a Healthcare Professional: Before starting any diet, especially one focused on managing a medical condition, it's crucial to consult with a healthcare professional or a registered dietitian.

Individual Variability: What works for one person may not work for another. The 21-day elimination diet is a tool for self-discovery and should be tailored to individual needs.

Long-Term Lifestyle Changes: The goal isn't just a short-term fix. The insights gained from the elimination diet can inform long-term dietary choices that support overall health and well-being for individuals with Hashimoto's disease.

Life after the elimination diet

Once you've completed the 21-day elimination diet for Hashimoto's and identified trigger foods, the focus shifts to creating a sustainable and healthy lifestyle. Here's what life might look like post-elimination diet:

1. **Personalized Diet:** Based on your experiences during the elimination diet, you now have a better understanding of which foods work well for you and which may trigger symptoms. This knowledge helps you shape a personalized, long-term eating plan.

2. **Balanced Nutrition:** Emphasize a well-rounded diet that includes a variety of nutrient-dense foods. Ensure you're getting enough vitamins, minerals, and other

essential nutrients to support overall health and thyroid function.

3. Regular Monitoring: Keep an eye on your symptoms and energy levels. Regular self-monitoring allows you to detect any patterns or signs of discomfort, helping you make necessary adjustments to your diet or lifestyle.

4. Mindful Eating: Cultivate a mindful approach to eating. Pay attention to how different foods make you feel and practice intuitive eating, listening to your body's cues about hunger and fullness.

5. Hydration: Stay well-hydrated. Water plays a crucial role in overall health, and proper hydration supports various bodily functions, including metabolism.

6. Stress Management: Stress can impact Hashimoto's symptoms, so adopting stress-management techniques such as meditation, deep breathing, or yoga can be beneficial.

7. Consistent Physical Activity: Integrate regular exercise into your daily schedule. Exercise not only supports weight management but also contributes to overall well-being and can help alleviate stress.

8. Consultation with Healthcare Professionals: Continue to work closely with healthcare professionals, including your doctor and a registered dietitian. Regular check-ups and discussions about your diet and symptoms ensure that you are on the right track.

9. Flexibility in Diet: While avoiding known trigger foods is important, it's also okay to be flexible. Occasional indulgences or trying new foods can be part of a balanced approach, as long as you remain mindful of how your body reacts.

10. Community Support: Connect with others who have Hashimoto's or autoimmune conditions. Sharing experiences, tips, and insights can provide valuable support and encouragement on your journey.

11. Educational Resources: Stay informed about Hashimoto's and autoimmune conditions. Knowledge is empowering, and understanding more about your condition helps you make informed choices about your health.

12. Celebrate Progress: Acknowledge and celebrate the progress you've made. Whether it's improved energy levels, better mood, or a clearer understanding of your body, recognizing achievements can boost motivation.

Remember, life after the elimination diet is about creating a sustainable and enjoyable lifestyle that supports your health and well-being. It's an ongoing journey of self-discovery, learning, and adapting to what works best for you.

CHAPTER 2: BREAKFAST

1. Mango Turmeric Lassi

INGREDIENTS

1 cup mango chunks (fresh or frozen)

1 cup plain Greek yogurt (or dairy-free alternative)

1/2 teaspoon turmeric powder

1 tablespoon honey or maple syrup

1/2 teaspoon ground ginger

1 cup water or coconut water

Ice cubes (optional)

PREPARATION

Blend all ingredients in a blender until smooth.

Add ice cubes if desired.

Pour into a glass and enjoy!

Prep Time: 5 minutes

Nutritional Value: Rich in probiotics, antioxidants, and anti-inflammatory properties.

2. Tahini Squash Porridge

INGREDIENTS

1 cup cooked butternut squash, mashed

2 tablespoons tahini

1 tablespoon chia seeds

1/2 teaspoon cinnamon

1/4 teaspoon nutmeg

1 cup almond milk (or any preferred milk)

PREPARATION

Combine mashed butternut squash, tahini, chia seeds, cinnamon, and nutmeg in a saucepan.

Heat over medium heat, stirring continuously.

Once heated, add almond milk and continue stirring until well combined and heated through.

Pour into a bowl and top with additional tahini if desired.

Prep Time: 10 minutes

Nutritional Value: High in fiber, healthy fats, and vitamins.

3. Veggie Scramble

INGREDIENTS

2 eggs (or tofu for a vegan option)

1/2 cup diced bell peppers

1/2 cup diced tomatoes

1/4 cup diced onions

1 cup spinach

Salt and pepper to taste

1 tablespoon olive oil

PREPARATION

Heat olive oil in a pan over medium heat.

Add onions and cook until translucent.

Add bell peppers and tomatoes, and sauté until softened.

Add spinach and cook until wilted.

Whisk eggs and pour them into the pan, stirring gently until cooked.

Season with salt and pepper.

Prep Time: 15 minutes

Nutritional Value: High in protein, vitamins, and minerals.

4. Bright Green Detox Smoothie

INGREDIENTS

1 cup kale leaves, stems removed

1/2 cucumber, peeled and sliced

1 green apple, cored and chopped

1/2 lemon, juiced

1-inch piece of ginger, peeled

1 cup coconut water

Ice cubes (optional)

PREPARATION

Blend all ingredients until smooth.

Add ice cubes if desired.

Pour into a glass and enjoy!

Prep Time: 5 minutes

Nutritional Value: Packed with antioxidants, vitamins, and hydration.

5. Red Velvet Smoothie

INGREDIENTS

1 small beet, peeled and diced

1 cup frozen mixed berries

1/2 cup Greek yogurt (or dairy-free alternative)

1 tablespoon cacao powder

1 tablespoon honey or maple syrup

1 cup almond milk

PREPARATION

Blend all ingredients until smooth.

Adjust sweetness with honey or maple syrup if needed.

Pour into a glass and enjoy!

Prep Time: 7 minutes

Nutritional Value: Rich in antioxidants, fiber, and probiotics.

6. Grain-Free Granola

INGREDIENTS

1 cup almonds, chopped

1 cup walnuts, chopped

1/2 cup unsweetened shredded coconut

1/4 cup chia seeds

1/4 cup coconut oil, melted

2 tablespoons honey or maple syrup

1 teaspoon vanilla extract

Pinch of salt

PREPARATION

Preheat the oven to 300°F (150°C).

In a bowl, mix almonds, walnuts, shredded coconut, and chia seeds.

In a separate bowl, mix melted coconut oil, honey or maple syrup, vanilla extract, and salt.

Combine wet and dry ingredients, and spread on a baking sheet.

Bake for 20-25 minutes or until golden brown, stirring occasionally.

Let it cool completely before storing.

Prep Time: 30 minutes

Nutritional Value: High in healthy fats, fiber, and protein.

7. Breakfast Sausage and Cauli-Hash

INGREDIENTS

1/2-pound breakfast sausage (choose a low-sugar option)

2 cups cauliflower rice

1/2 onion, diced

1 bell pepper, diced

2 tablespoons olive oil

Salt and pepper to taste

PREPARATION

In a skillet, cook the sausage until browned. Remove and set aside.

In the same skillet, add olive oil, onions, and bell peppers. Cook until softened.

Add cauliflower rice and cooked sausage, and cook until cauliflower is tender.

Season with salt and pepper to taste.

Prep Time: 20 minutes

Nutritional Value: Low-carb and high in protein.

8. Banana-Walnut Almond Flour Muffins

INGREDIENTS

2 ripe bananas, mashed

3 eggs

1/4 cup coconut oil, melted

1 teaspoon vanilla extract

2 cups almond flour

1/2 teaspoon baking soda

1/4 teaspoon salt

1/2 cup chopped walnuts

PREPARATION

Preheat the oven to 350°F (175°C). Line a muffin tin with paper liners.

In a bowl, mix mashed bananas, eggs melted coconut oil, and vanilla extract.

In a separate bowl, combine almond flour, baking soda, and salt.

Gradually add the dry ingredients to the wet ingredients, mixing well.

Fold in chopped walnuts.

Spoon the batter into muffin cups and bake for 20-25 minutes or until a toothpick comes out clean.

Prep Time: 30 minutes

Nutritional Value: Gluten-free and high in healthy fats.

9. Spinach and Herb Frittata

INGREDIENTS

6 eggs

1 cup fresh spinach, chopped

1/2 cup fresh herbs (such as parsley, chives, or dill), chopped

1/2 cup cherry tomatoes, halved

Salt and pepper to taste

1 tablespoon olive oil

PREPARATION

Preheat the oven to 350°F (175°C).

In a bowl, whisk eggs and season with salt and pepper.

Heat olive oil in an oven-safe skillet over medium heat.

Add spinach, herbs, and tomatoes to the skillet, and sauté until spinach wilts.

Pour the whisked eggs over the vegetables in the skillet.

Cook for a few minutes until the edges start to set.

Transfer the skillet to the oven and bake for 15-20 minutes or until the frittata is set and slightly golden.

Prep Time: 25 minutes

Nutritional Value: High in protein, vitamins, and minerals.

10.   Raspberry Cinnamon Yogurt Bowl

INGREDIENTS

1 cup plain Greek yogurt (or dairy-free alternative)

1/2 cup fresh raspberries

1 tablespoon chia seeds

1 tablespoon almond butter

1/2 teaspoon cinnamon

1 teaspoon honey or maple syrup (optional)

PREPARATION

In a bowl, layer Greek yogurt, fresh raspberries, and chia seeds.

Drizzle with almond butter and sprinkle with cinnamon.

Add honey or maple syrup if desired.

Prep Time: 5 minutes

Nutritional Value: High in protein, fiber, and antioxidants.

11.   Apple-Carrot Breakfast Muffins

INGREDIENTS

1 cup almond flour

1/2 cup coconut flour

1 teaspoon baking soda

1/2 teaspoon cinnamon

Pinch of salt

2 eggs

1/4 cup coconut oil, melted

1/4 cup honey or maple syrup

1 cup grated apples

1 cup grated carrots

PREPARATION

Preheat the oven to 350°F (175°C). Line a muffin tin with paper liners.

In a bowl, whisk together almond flour, coconut flour, baking soda, cinnamon, and salt.

In another bowl, beat eggs and mix in melted coconut oil and honey or maple syrup.

Gradually add the wet ingredients to the dry ingredients, stirring until well combined.

Fold in grated apples and carrots.

Spoon the batter into muffin cups and bake for 20-25 minutes or until a toothpick comes out clean.

Prep Time: 30 minutes

Nutritional Value: Gluten-free and high in fiber.

12. Fruit and Coconut Yogurt Parfait

INGREDIENTS

1 cup coconut yogurt

1/2 cup mixed berries (strawberries, blueberries, raspberries)

1/4 cup granola (choose a gluten-free option if needed)

1 tablespoon shredded coconut

Drizzle of honey or maple syrup (optional)

Preparation:

In a glass or bowl, layer coconut yogurt, mixed berries, and granola.

Repeat the layers until the container is filled.

Top with shredded coconut.

Drizzle with honey or maple syrup if desired.

Prep Time: 5 minutes

Nutritional Value: High in probiotics, antioxidants, and fiber.

CHAPTER 3: SNACKS AND TREATS

1. Homemade Cherry Gummies

INGREDIENTS

1 cup cherry juice (unsweetened)

3 tablespoons grass-fed gelatin

1-2 tablespoons honey or maple syrup (optional)

PREPARATION

Heat cherry juice in a saucepan over low heat.

Gradually whisk in gelatin until fully dissolved.

If using, add honey or maple syrup and stir until well combined.

Pour the mixture into silicone molds or a shallow dish.

Refrigerate for at least 2 hours or until set.

Pop out of the molds or cut into squares.

Prep Time: 10 minutes + chilling time

Nutritional Value: Rich in antioxidants and gut-friendly gelatin.

2.   Strawberry Fruit Tart

INGREDIENTS

For the crust:

1 cup almond flour

1/4 cup coconut oil, melted

2 tablespoons honey or maple syrup

For the filling:

1 cup coconut cream

1 teaspoon vanilla extract

Fresh strawberries, sliced

PREPARATION

Preheat the oven to 350°F (175°C).

Mix almond flour, melted coconut oil, and honey or maple syrup for the crust.

Press the mixture into a tart pan and bake for 10-12 minutes or until golden brown. Let it cool.

Whip coconut cream with vanilla extract until fluffy.

Spread the coconut cream over the cooled crust.

Arrange sliced strawberries on top.

Refrigerate for at least 1 hour before serving.

Prep Time: 20 minutes + chilling time

Nutritional Value: High in healthy fats and antioxidants.

3. Slow Cooker Poached Pears

INGREDIENTS

4 ripe but firm pears, peeled and cored

1 cup water

1/2 cup honey or maple syrup

1 cinnamon stick

4 cloves

1 teaspoon vanilla extract

PREPARATION

Place pears in the slow cooker.

In a bowl, mix water, honey or maple syrup, cinnamon stick, cloves, and vanilla extract.

Pour the mixture over the pears.

Cook on low for 2-3 hours or until the pears are tender.

Serve warm, drizzled with the poaching liquid.

Prep Time: 10 minutes + slow cooking time

Nutritional Value: Rich in fiber, vitamins, and minerals.

4.   Spiced Walnuts

INGREDIENTS

1 cup raw walnuts

1 tablespoon coconut oil, melted

1 teaspoon cinnamon

1/2 teaspoon ground ginger

Pinch of sea salt

1 tablespoon maple syrup (optional)

PREPARATION

Preheat the oven to 350°F (175°C).

In a bowl, toss walnuts with melted coconut oil, cinnamon, ground ginger, and salt.

Spread the walnuts on a baking sheet.

Bake for 10-12 minutes, stirring halfway through.

If using, drizzle maple syrup over the walnuts and toss to coat.

Let them cool completely before serving.

Prep Time: 15 minutes

Nutritional Value: High in healthy fats and antioxidants.

5.   Avocado Deviled Eggs

INGREDIENTS

6 hard-boiled eggs, halved

1 ripe avocado, mashed

1 tablespoon lemon juice

1 teaspoon Dijon mustard

Salt and pepper to taste

Paprika for garnish

PREPARATION

Remove yolks from eggs and place them in a bowl.

Add mashed avocado, lemon juice, Dijon mustard, salt, and pepper to the yolks.

Mash and mix until smooth.

Spoon the mixture into the egg whites.

Sprinkle with paprika for garnish.

Prep Time: 15 minutes

Nutritional Value: High in healthy fats and protein.

6. Crispy, Crunchy Carrot Fries

INGREDIENTS

4 large carrots, peeled and cut into matchsticks

1 tablespoon olive oil

1 teaspoon paprika

1/2 teaspoon garlic powder

Salt and pepper to taste

PREPARATION

Preheat the oven to 425°F (220°C).

In a bowl, toss carrot matchsticks with olive oil, paprika, garlic powder, salt, and pepper.

Spread the carrots on a baking sheet in a single layer.

Bake for 20-25 minutes or until crispy, stirring halfway through.

Prep Time: 15 minutes

Nutritional Value: High in fiber, vitamins, and antioxidants.

7.   Kale Chips

INGREDIENTS

1 bunch kale, stems removed and torn into bite-sized pieces

1 tablespoon olive oil

1/2 teaspoon sea salt

1/4 teaspoon garlic powder

1/4 teaspoon paprika

PREPARATION

Preheat the oven to 350°F (175°C).

In a bowl, toss kale pieces with olive oil, sea salt, garlic powder, and paprika.

Spread the kale on a baking sheet.

Bake for 10-15 minutes or until crispy, checking frequently to prevent burning.

Prep Time: 15 minutes

Nutritional Value: High in fiber, vitamins, and minerals.

8.   Guacamole with Jicama

INGREDIENTS

3 ripe avocados, peeled and mashed

1/4 cup red onion, finely diced

1/4 cup fresh cilantro, chopped

1 jalapeño, seeded and minced

1 lime, juiced

Salt and pepper to taste

Jicama sticks for dipping

PREPARATION

In a bowl, combine mashed avocados, red onion, cilantro, jalapeño, lime juice, salt, and pepper.

Mix until well combined.

Serve with jicama sticks for dipping.

Prep Time: 15 minutes

Nutritional Value: High in healthy fats, fiber, and vitamins.

9. Zucchini Rounds with Tapenade

INGREDIENTS

2 zucchini, sliced into rounds

1 tablespoon olive oil

Salt and pepper to taste

Olive tapenade for topping

PREPARATION

Preheat the oven to 400°F (200°C).

Toss zucchini rounds with olive oil, salt, and pepper.

Arrange the rounds on a baking sheet.

Bake for 15-20 minutes or until golden brown.

Top each round with a small dollop of olive tapenade.

Prep Time: 20 minutes

Nutritional Value: Low-carb and high in fiber.

10. Refrigerator Dill Pickles

INGREDIENTS

4-5 small cucumbers, sliced

1 cup water

1 cup white vinegar

1 tablespoon salt

1 tablespoon dill seeds

1 teaspoon black peppercorns

2 cloves garlic, minced

PREPARATION

In a jar, combine water, white vinegar, salt, dill seeds, black peppercorns, and minced garlic.

Stir until the salt dissolves.

Add cucumber slices to the jar, ensuring they are fully submerged in the liquid.

Seal the jar and refrigerate for at least 24 hours before serving.

Prep Time: 10 minutes + chilling time

Nutritional Value: Low-calorie and a source of probiotics.

11. Plantain Chips

INGREDIENTS

2 green plantains, thinly sliced

2 tablespoons coconut oil, melted

Salt to taste

Preparation:

Preheat the oven to 375°F (190°C).

Toss plantain slices with melted coconut oil and salt.

Arrange the slices on a baking sheet.

Bake for 15-20 minutes or until crispy, flipping halfway through.

Prep Time: 15 minutes

Nutritional Value: High in fiber and a healthier alternative to traditional chips.

12. Cherry Tiger-nut Flour Leather

INGREDIENTS

2 cups cherries, pitted

1/2 cup tiger nut flour

2 tablespoons honey or maple syrup

PREPARATION

Preheat the oven to 170°F (75°C) or the lowest setting.

In a blender, puree cherries until smooth.

In a bowl, combine cherry puree, tiger nut flour, and honey or maple syrup.

Spread the mixture onto a parchment-lined baking sheet.

Dehydrate in the oven for 6-8 hours or until the leather is no longer sticky.

Cut into strips and roll up.

Prep Time: 15 minutes + dehydrating time

Nutritional Value: High in antioxidants and a healthy alternative to commercial fruit leather.

CHAPTER 4: EASY VEGETABLES AND SIDES

1. Cold Asian Zoodle Salad

INGREDIENTS

2 medium zucchinis, spiralized

1 carrot, julienned

1/2 cup red cabbage, thinly sliced

1/4 cup chopped scallions

1/4 cup chopped cilantro

2 tablespoons sesame oil

2 tablespoons tamari or coconut aminos

1 tablespoon rice vinegar

1 tablespoon sesame seeds (optional)

PREPARATION

In a large bowl, combine zucchini noodles, julienned carrot, sliced red cabbage, scallions, and cilantro.

In a small bowl, whisk together sesame oil, tamari or coconut aminos, and rice vinegar.

Pour the dressing over the vegetables and toss until well coated.

Sprinkle with sesame seeds if desired.

Refrigerate for at least 30 minutes before serving.

Prep Time: 15 minutes

Nutritional Value: Low-carb, high in fiber, and antioxidants.

2.   Baked Herbed Zucchini Boats

INGREDIENTS

4 medium zucchinis, halved lengthwise

1 tablespoon olive oil

1 cup cherry tomatoes, halved

1/2 cup feta cheese, crumbled

2 tablespoons fresh basil, chopped

Salt and pepper to taste

PREPARATION

Preheat the oven to 375°F (190°C).

Scoop out the centers of the zucchini halves, leaving a boat-like shape.

Brush the zucchini with olive oil and place them in a baking dish.

In a bowl, mix cherry tomatoes, feta cheese, and fresh basil. Season with salt and pepper.

Spoon the mixture into the zucchini boats.

Bake for 20-25 minutes or until the zucchini is tender.

Prep Time: 15 minutes

Nutritional Value: Low-carb, high in fiber, and a good source of vitamins and minerals.

3. Creamy Pineapple Coleslaw

INGREDIENTS

4 cups shredded cabbage

1 cup shredded carrots

1 cup pineapple chunks

1/2 cup mayonnaise (preferably homemade or a quality store-bought)

2 tablespoons apple cider vinegar

1 tablespoon honey or maple syrup

Salt and pepper to taste

PREPARATION

In a large bowl, combine shredded cabbage, shredded carrots, and pineapple chunks.

In a small bowl, whisk together mayonnaise, apple cider vinegar, honey or maple syrup, salt, and pepper.

Pour the dressing over the coleslaw and toss until well-coated.

Refrigerate for at least 1 hour before serving.

Prep Time: 15 minutes

Nutritional Value: Rich in fiber, vitamins, and natural sweetness from pineapple.

4. Stuffed Zucchini

INGREDIENTS

4 medium zucchinis, halved lengthwise

1 tablespoon olive oil

1 onion, diced

2 cloves garlic, minced

1 bell pepper, diced

1 cup cherry tomatoes, halved

1 cup spinach, chopped

1/2 cup feta cheese, crumbled

Salt and pepper to taste

PREPARATION

Preheat the oven to 375°F (190°C).

Scoop out the centers of the zucchini halves.

In a pan, heat olive oil over medium heat. Add onion and garlic, and sauté until softened.

Add bell pepper, cherry tomatoes, and spinach. Cook until the vegetables are tender.

Fill the zucchini halves with the vegetable mixture.

Top with crumbled feta cheese.

Bake for 20-25 minutes or until the zucchini is cooked through.

Prep Time: 25 minutes

Nutritional Value: Low-carb, high in fiber, and a good source of vitamins.

5.   Veggie "Rice" Bowl

INGREDIENTS

2 cups cauliflower rice

1 tablespoon coconut oil

1 cup broccoli florets

1 carrot, grated

1/2 cup snap peas, sliced

2 tablespoons tamari or coconut aminos

1 teaspoon sesame oil

1 tablespoon sesame seeds (optional)

Chopped green onions for garnish

PREPARATION

In a food processor, pulse cauliflower until it resembles rice.

In a pan, heat coconut oil over medium heat. Add cauliflower rice and cook until tender.

Add broccoli, grated carrot, and snap peas. Cook until the vegetables are crisp-tender.

In a small bowl, mix tamari or coconut aminos with sesame oil. Pour over the vegetable rice mixture.

Toss until well combined. Garnish with sesame seeds and chopped green onions.

Prep Time: 20 minutes

Nutritional Value: Low-carb, low-calorie, and high in fiber.

6. Spaghetti Squash Marinara

INGREDIENTS

1 medium spaghetti squash

2 tablespoons olive oil

1 onion, diced

2 cloves garlic, minced

1 can (14 oz) crushed tomatoes

1 teaspoon dried oregano

1 teaspoon dried basil

Salt and pepper to taste

Fresh parsley for garnish

PREPARATION

Preheat the oven to 375°F (190°C).

Cut the spaghetti squash in half lengthwise and remove the seeds.

Drizzle with olive oil and place the squash, cut side down, on a baking sheet.

Bake for 40-45 minutes or until the squash is fork-tender.

In a pan, heat olive oil over medium heat. Add onion and garlic, and sauté until softened.

Add crushed tomatoes, oregano, basil, salt, and pepper. Simmer for 15-20 minutes.

Scrape the spaghetti squash with a fork to create "noodles."

Top with marinara sauce and garnish with fresh parsley.

Prep Time: 50 minutes

Nutritional Value: Low-carb, high in fiber, and a good source of vitamins.

7.   Huevos Rancheros

INGREDIENTS

4 eggs

1 tablespoon olive oil

1 onion, diced

2 cloves garlic, minced

1 bell pepper, diced

1 can (14 oz) diced tomatoes

1 teaspoon ground cumin

1 teaspoon chili powder

Salt and pepper to taste

Fresh cilantro for garnish

Avocado slices for serving

PREPARATION

In a pan, heat olive oil over medium heat. Add onion and garlic, and sauté until softened.

Add bell pepper, diced tomatoes, ground cumin, chili powder, salt, and pepper. Simmer for 10 minutes.

Make wells in the tomato mixture and crack eggs into each well.

Cover and cook until the eggs are cooked to your liking.

Garnish with fresh cilantro and serve with avocado slices.

Prep Time: 20 minutes

Nutritional Value: High in protein, vitamins, and healthy fats.

8.   Sweet Potato Curry

INGREDIENTS

2 medium sweet potatoes, peeled and diced

1 tablespoon coconut oil

1 onion, diced

2 cloves garlic, minced

1 tablespoon grated ginger

1 tablespoon curry powder

1 can (14 oz) coconut milk

1 cup vegetable broth

1 cup spinach

Salt and pepper to taste

Fresh cilantro for garnish

PREPARATION

In a pot, heat coconut oil over medium heat. Add onion, garlic, and grated ginger, and sauté until softened.

Add curry powder and stir for 1-2 minutes.

Add diced sweet potatoes, coconut milk, and vegetable broth. Bring to a simmer and cook until sweet potatoes are tender.

Stir in spinach until wilted.

Season with salt and pepper. Garnish with fresh cilantro.

Prep Time: 30 minutes

Nutritional Value: High in fiber, vitamins, and anti-inflammatory properties.

9. Balsamic Marinated Fennel Salad

INGREDIENTS

2 fennel bulbs, thinly sliced

1/4 cup olive oil

2 tablespoons balsamic vinegar

1 teaspoon Dijon mustard

1 teaspoon honey or maple syrup

Salt and pepper to taste

Chopped fresh parsley for garnish

PREPARATION

In a bowl, whisk together olive oil, balsamic vinegar, Dijon mustard, honey or maple syrup, salt, and pepper.

Add thinly sliced fennel to the bowl and toss until well coated.

Let it marinate for at least 30 minutes.

Garnish with chopped fresh parsley before serving.

Prep Time: 15 minutes + marinating time

Nutritional Value: Low-calorie, high in fiber, and a good source of vitamins.

10. Quick Pickled Red Onions

INGREDIENTS

1 large red onion, thinly sliced

1/2 cup apple cider vinegar

1 tablespoon honey or maple syrup

1 teaspoon salt

1/2 teaspoon black peppercorns

1 bay leaf

PREPARATION

Place the thinly sliced red onion in a jar.

In a small saucepan, combine apple cider vinegar, honey or maple syrup, salt, black peppercorns, and bay leaf.

Bring the mixture to a simmer, stirring until the salt dissolves.

Pour the hot liquid over the red onions in the jar.

Allow the pickled onions to cool to room temperature before sealing the jar.

Refrigerate for at least 1 hour before serving.

Prep Time: 15 minutes + pickling time

Nutritional Value: Low-calorie, adds flavor to dishes, and is a source of probiotics.

CHAPTER 5: MAIN SEAFOODS

1. Mahi-Mahi with Mango Agrodolce

INGREDIENTS

4 mahi-mahi fillets

Salt and pepper to taste

1 tablespoon olive oil

For Mango Agrodolce:

1 ripe mango, peeled and diced

2 tablespoons balsamic vinegar

1 tablespoon honey or maple syrup

1 teaspoon grated ginger

Salt to taste

PREPARATION

Season mahi-mahi fillets with salt and pepper.

In a skillet, heat olive oil over medium-high heat.

Pan-sear the mahi-mahi fillets for 3-4 minutes per side or until cooked through.

In a separate saucepan, combine diced mango, balsamic vinegar, honey or maple syrup, grated ginger, and salt.

Simmer over medium heat until the mango is softened and the sauce is slightly thickened.

Serve the mahi-mahi fillets topped with mango agrodolce.

Prep Time: 20 minutes

Nutritional Value: High in omega-3 fatty acids, protein, and vitamins.

2.   Pan-Roasted Halibut

INGREDIENTS

4 halibut fillets

2 tablespoons olive oil

Salt and pepper to taste

1 lemon, sliced

Fresh herbs for garnish (such as parsley or dill)

PREPARATION

Preheat the oven to 400°F (200°C).

Season halibut fillets with salt and pepper.

In an oven-safe skillet, heat olive oil over medium-high heat.

Sear the halibut fillets for 2 minutes on each side.

Place lemon slices on top of each fillet.

Transfer the skillet to the preheated oven and roast for 8-10 minutes or until the halibut is cooked through.

Garnish with fresh herbs before serving.

Prep Time: 15 minutes

Nutritional Value: High in protein, omega-3 fatty acids, and vitamin D.

3.   Mexican Cod Fish Tacos

INGREDIENTS

1 lb cod fillets

1 tablespoon olive oil

1 teaspoon chili powder

1/2 teaspoon cumin

1/2 teaspoon paprika

Salt and pepper to taste

Corn or gluten-free tortillas

Cabbage slaw (shredded cabbage, lime juice, and cilantro) for topping

Salsa and avocado slices for serving

PREPARATION

Preheat the oven to 375°F (190°C).

In a bowl, mix olive oil, chili powder, cumin, paprika, salt, and pepper.

Brush the cod fillets with the spice mixture.

Bake for 12-15 minutes or until the cod is flaky.

Flake the cod and assemble tacos with tortillas, cabbage slaw, salsa, and avocado slices.

Prep Time: 20 minutes

Nutritional Value: High in protein, fiber, and healthy fats.

4. Ginger-Spiced Tuna Salad Wraps

INGREDIENTS

2 cans (5 oz each) tuna, drained

1/4 cup mayonnaise (preferably homemade or a quality store-bought)

1 tablespoon grated ginger

1 tablespoon soy sauce or tamari

1 teaspoon sesame oil

Lettuce leaves or gluten-free wraps

Avocado slices and cucumber strips for topping

PREPARATION

In a bowl, mix drained tuna, mayonnaise, grated ginger, soy sauce or tamari, and sesame oil.

Spoon the tuna mixture onto lettuce leaves or wraps.

Top with avocado slices and cucumber strips.

Roll into wraps and secure with toothpicks if needed.

Prep Time: 15 minutes

Nutritional Value: High in protein, omega-3 fatty acids, and antioxidants.

5.   Shrimp Curry

INGREDIENTS

1 lb shrimp, peeled and deveined

1 tablespoon coconut oil

1 onion, finely chopped

2 cloves garlic, minced

1 tablespoon grated ginger

1 tablespoon curry powder

1 can (14 oz) coconut milk

1 cup cherry tomatoes, halved

Fresh cilantro for garnish

Salt and pepper to taste

PREPARATION

In a pan, heat coconut oil over medium heat. Add chopped onion, minced garlic, and grated ginger. Sauté until softened.

Add curry powder and stir for 1-2 minutes.

Add peeled and deveined shrimp, and cook until they turn pink.

Pour in coconut milk and add cherry tomatoes. Simmer for 5-7 minutes.

Season with salt and pepper. Garnish with fresh cilantro before serving.

Prep Time: 25 minutes

Nutritional Value: High in protein, healthy fats, and anti-inflammatory spices.

6.   Shrimp Cauliflower Fried Rice

INGREDIENTS

1 lb shrimp, peeled and deveined

1 head cauliflower, grated

2 tablespoons coconut oil

1 onion, diced

2 carrots, diced

2 cloves garlic, minced

1 tablespoon grated ginger

2 eggs, beaten

3 tablespoons tamari or coconut aminos

Green onions for garnish

Sesame seeds for garnish

PREPARATION

In a pan, heat coconut oil over medium heat. Add diced onion, carrots, minced garlic, and grated ginger. Sauté until vegetables are tender.

Push the vegetables to one side of the pan and pour the beaten eggs into the other side. Scramble the eggs until cooked.

Add grated cauliflower to the pan and stir-fry for 3-4 minutes.

Add peeled and deveined shrimp, and cook until they turn pink.

Pour tamari or coconut aminos over the mixture and stir to combine.

Garnish with green onions and sesame seeds before serving.

Prep Time: 30 minutes

Nutritional Value: Low-carb, high in protein, and a good source of vitamins.

7. White Fish Red Curry

INGREDIENTS

4 white fish fillets (such as tilapia or cod)

1 tablespoon red curry paste

1 can (14 oz) coconut milk

1 red bell pepper, sliced

1 zucchini, sliced

1 tablespoon fish sauce

Fresh basil leaves for garnish

Cooked rice for serving

PREPARATION

In a pan, heat red curry paste over medium heat for 1-2 minutes.

Pour in coconut milk and stir until the curry paste is fully dissolved.

Add sliced red bell pepper and zucchini to the pan. Simmer for 5-7 minutes.

Season fish fillets with salt and pepper, then add them to the pan.

Cook for 5-7 minutes or until the fish is cooked through.

Stir in fish sauce and garnish with fresh basil.

Serve over cooked rice.

Prep Time: 25 minutes

Nutritional Value: High in protein, healthy fats, and anti-inflammatory properties.

8.   Poached   Cod   with Summer Vegetables and Quinoa

INGREDIENTS

4 cod fillets

1 tablespoon olive oil

1 onion, diced

2 cloves garlic, minced

1 zucchini, diced

1 yellow squash, diced

1 cup cherry tomatoes, halved

1 cup quinoa, cooked

Fresh parsley for garnish

Lemon wedges for serving

Salt and pepper to taste

PREPARATION

Season cod fillets with salt and pepper.

In a large skillet, heat olive oil over medium heat. Add diced onion and minced garlic, and sauté until softened.

Add diced zucchini and yellow squash, and cook until tender.

Place cod fillets on top of the vegetable mixture and add cherry tomatoes.

Cover the skillet and poach the cod for 8-10 minutes or until it flakes easily.

Serve the cod over cooked quinoa, garnished with fresh parsley and lemon wedges.

Prep Time: 30 minutes

Nutritional Value: High in protein, fiber, and vitamins.

9. Spicy Shrimp, Okra, and Tomato Stew

INGREDIENTS

1 lb shrimp, peeled and deveined

2 tablespoons olive oil

1 onion, diced

2 cloves garlic, minced

1 teaspoon smoked paprika

1/2 teaspoon cayenne pepper

1 can (14 oz) diced tomatoes

1 cup okra, sliced

Salt and pepper to taste

Fresh cilantro for garnish

PREPARATION

In a pan, heat olive oil over medium heat. Add diced onion and minced garlic, and sauté until softened.

Add smoked paprika and cayenne pepper, and stir for 1-2 minutes.

Add peeled and deveined shrimp, and cook until they turn pink.

Pour in diced tomatoes and sliced okra. Simmer for 10-12 minutes.

Season with salt and pepper. Garnish with fresh cilantro before serving.

Prep Time: 25 minutes

Nutritional Value: High in protein, antioxidants, and anti-inflammatory spices.

10. Crab and Asparagus Casserole

INGREDIENTS

1 lb crab meat

1 lb asparagus, trimmed and blanched

1/4 cup mayonnaise (preferably homemade or a quality store-bought)

1/4 cup sour cream

1 tablespoon Dijon mustard

1 teaspoon Old Bay seasoning

1 cup shredded cheddar cheese

Chopped chives for garnish

PREPARATION

Preheat the oven to 375°F (190°C).

In a bowl, combine crab meat, blanched asparagus, mayonnaise, sour cream, Dijon mustard, and Old Bay seasoning.

Transfer the mixture to a baking dish.

Top with shredded cheddar cheese.

Bake for 20-25 minutes or until the casserole is bubbly and the cheese is melted.

Garnish with chopped chives before serving.

Prep Time: 30 minutes

Nutritional Value: High in protein, healthy fats, and vitamins.

CHAPTER 6: POULTRY AND MEAT

1. Nutty Chicken Lettuce Wraps

INGREDIENTS

1 lb ground chicken

1 tablespoon coconut oil

1/2 cup water chestnuts, chopped

1/4 cup green onions, sliced

2 tablespoons almond butter

1 tablespoon coconut aminos

1 teaspoon sesame oil

Butter lettuce leaves for wrapping

PREPARATION

In a skillet, heat coconut oil over medium heat. Add ground chicken and cook until browned.

Add water chestnuts and green onions to the skillet. Cook for an additional 2-3 minutes.

In a small bowl, mix almond butter, coconut aminos, and sesame oil. Pour over the chicken mixture and stir to combine.

Spoon the mixture into butter lettuce leaves for wraps.

Prep Time: 20 minutes

Nutritional Value: High in protein, healthy fats, and low in carbs.

2.   Lamb Shepherd's Pie

INGREDIENTS

1 lb ground lamb

1 onion, diced

2 carrots, diced

2 cloves garlic, minced

1 cup green peas

1 cup beef or vegetable broth

2 tablespoons tomato paste

2 tablespoons butter or ghee

4 cups cauliflower florets

Salt and pepper to taste

PREPARATION

Preheat the oven to 400°F (200°C).

In a skillet, brown ground lamb over medium heat. Add diced onion, carrots, and minced garlic. Cook until vegetables are tender.

Stir in green peas, beef or vegetable broth, and tomato paste. Simmer for 10-12 minutes.

In a separate pot, steam cauliflower until tender. Mash with butter or ghee, and season with salt and pepper.

Transfer the lamb mixture to a baking dish and top with mashed cauliflower.

Bake for 20-25 minutes or until the top is golden.

Prep Time: 45 minutes

Nutritional Value: High in protein, healthy fats, and low in carbs.

3.   Creamy Beef Casserole

INGREDIENTS

1.5 lbs ground beef

1 onion, diced

2 cloves garlic, minced

1 cup mushrooms, sliced

1 cup spinach, chopped

1 cup coconut milk

1/4 cup nutritional yeast

Salt and pepper to taste

PREPARATION

Preheat the oven to 375°F (190°C).

In a skillet, brown ground beef over medium heat. Add diced onion, minced garlic, mushrooms, and spinach. Cook until vegetables are tender.

In a bowl, mix coconut milk and nutritional yeast. Pour over the beef mixture and stir to combine.

Transfer the mixture to a baking dish.

Bake for 20-25 minutes or until the casserole is bubbly.

Prep Time: 35 minutes

Nutritional Value: High in protein, healthy fats, and dairy-free.

4. Turkey Piccata with Lemon Zucchini

INGREDIENTS

1.5 lbs turkey breast, sliced thin

Salt and pepper to taste

2 tablespoons coconut flour

2 tablespoons coconut oil

1/2 cup chicken broth

Juice of 2 lemons

2 tablespoons capers

2 zucchinis, spiralized

Fresh parsley for garnish

PREPARATION

Season turkey slices with salt and pepper, then dredge in coconut flour.

In a skillet, heat coconut oil over medium-high heat. Cook turkey slices for 2-3 minutes per side until golden.

Remove the turkey from the skillet. In the same skillet, add chicken broth, lemon juice, and capers. Simmer for 5 minutes.

In a separate pan, sauté spiralized zucchini until tender.

Serve turkey over lemon zucchini, drizzle with piccata sauce, and garnish with fresh parsley.

Prep Time: 25 minutes

Nutritional Value: High in protein, low-carb, and a good source of vitamins.

5.   Slow Cooker Sloppy Joe Bowls

INGREDIENTS

2 lbs ground beef

1 onion, diced

2 cloves garlic, minced

1 bell pepper, diced

1 can (14 oz) crushed tomatoes

1/4 cup tomato paste

2 tablespoons apple cider vinegar

1 tablespoon honey or maple syrup

1 teaspoon chili powder

Salt and pepper to taste

Sweet potato or cauliflower rice for serving

PREPARATION

In a skillet, brown ground beef over medium heat. Add diced onion, minced garlic, and bell pepper. Cook until vegetables are tender.

Transfer the beef mixture to a slow cooker.

Add crushed tomatoes, tomato paste, apple cider vinegar, honey or maple syrup, chili powder, salt, and pepper. Stir to combine.

Cook on low for 4-6 hours.

Serve over sweet potato or cauliflower rice.

Prep Time: 20 minutes (plus slow cooker time)

Nutritional Value: High in protein, low-carb, and free from refined sugars.

6. Steak Fajitas with Onions and Peppers

INGREDIENTS

1.5 lbs flank steak, sliced thin

1 onion, sliced

2 bell peppers, sliced

2 tablespoons olive oil

1 tablespoon chili powder

1 teaspoon cumin

1 teaspoon smoked paprika

Salt and pepper to taste

Lettuce leaves or gluten-free tortillas for serving

Guacamole and salsa for topping

PREPARATION

In a bowl, mix sliced flank steak, sliced onion, sliced bell peppers, olive oil, chili powder, cumin, smoked paprika, salt, and pepper.

Heat a skillet over medium-high heat. Add the steak and vegetable mixture. Cook for 8-10 minutes until steak is cooked and vegetables are tender.

Serve the fajita mixture in lettuce leaves or gluten-free tortillas.

Top with guacamole and salsa.

Prep Time: 30 minutes

Nutritional Value: High in protein, low-carb, and a good source of vitamins.

7. Cucumber Salad

INGREDIENTS

2 cucumbers, thinly sliced

1/4 cup red onion, thinly sliced

1/4 cup fresh dill, chopped

2 tablespoons apple cider vinegar

1 tablespoon olive oil

Salt and pepper to taste

PREPARATION

In a bowl, combine thinly sliced cucumbers, thinly sliced red onion, and chopped fresh dill.

In a small bowl, whisk together apple cider vinegar, olive oil, salt, and pepper.

Pour the dressing over the cucumber mixture and toss until well-coated.

Refrigerate for at least 30 minutes before serving.

Prep Time: 10 minutes

Nutritional Value: Low-calorie, hydrating, and a good source of vitamins.

8. Meatloaf Meatballs Lettuce Wraps with Dipping Sauce

INGREDIENTS

For Meatballs:

1 lb ground beef

1 egg

1/2 cup almond flour

1/4 cup almond milk

2 tablespoons tomato paste

1 teaspoon garlic powder

1 teaspoon onion powder

Salt and pepper to taste

For Dipping Sauce:

1/4 cup mayonnaise (preferably homemade or a quality store-bought)

1 tablespoon Dijon mustard

1 tablespoon honey or maple syrup

PREPARATION

Preheat the oven to 375°F (190°C).

In a bowl, combine ground beef, egg, almond flour, almond milk, tomato paste, garlic powder, onion powder, salt, and pepper.

Shape the mixture into meatballs and place them on a baking sheet.

Bake for 20-25 minutes or until the meatballs are cooked through.

In a small bowl, whisk together mayonnaise, Dijon mustard, and honey or maple syrup to make the dipping sauce.

Serve meatballs in lettuce wraps with the dipping sauce.

Prep Time: 30 minutes

Nutritional Value: High in protein, low-carb, and gluten-free.

9.   Unstuffed Cabbage Rolls

INGREDIENTS

1 lb ground turkey

1 onion, diced

2 cloves garlic, minced

1 cabbage, shredded

1 can (14 oz) diced tomatoes

1 can (14 oz) tomato sauce

1 teaspoon dried oregano

1 teaspoon dried thyme

Salt and pepper to taste

PREPARATION

In a skillet, brown ground turkey over medium heat. Add diced onion and minced garlic. Cook until onion is translucent.

Add shredded cabbage, diced tomatoes, tomato sauce, dried oregano, dried thyme, salt, and pepper. Stir to combine.

Simmer for 15-20 minutes until the cabbage is tender.

Prep Time: 30 minutes

Nutritional Value: High in protein, low-carb, and a good source of fiber.

10. Cinnamon Lamb Skillet

INGREDIENTS

1.5 lbs ground lamb

1 onion, diced

2 cloves garlic, minced

1 teaspoon ground cinnamon

1 teaspoon cumin

1 teaspoon coriander

1 cup cherry tomatoes, halved

Fresh mint for garnish

Salt and pepper to taste

PREPARATION

In a skillet, brown ground lamb over medium heat. Add diced onion and minced garlic. Cook until onion is translucent.

Stir in ground cinnamon, cumin, coriander, salt, and pepper.

Add cherry tomatoes and cook for an additional 5 minutes.

Garnish with fresh mint before serving.

Prep Time: 25 minutes

Nutritional Value: High in protein, rich in aromatic spices, and low in carbs.

11. Mediterranean Chicken Pizzas

INGREDIENTS

4 boneless, skinless chicken breasts

2 tablespoons olive oil

1 teaspoon dried oregano

1 teaspoon dried basil

1/2 teaspoon garlic powder

Salt and pepper to taste

1 cup cherry tomatoes, sliced

1/2 cup black olives, sliced

1/2 cup feta cheese, crumbled

Fresh basil for garnish

PREPARATION

Preheat the oven to 400°F (200°C).

Place chicken breasts on a baking sheet. Drizzle with olive oil and sprinkle with dried oregano, dried basil, garlic powder, salt, and pepper.

Bake for 20-25 minutes or until the chicken is cooked through.

Top each chicken breast with sliced cherry tomatoes, sliced black olives, and crumbled feta cheese.

Return to the oven and bake for an additional 5 minutes or until the cheese is melted.

Garnish with fresh basil before serving.

Prep Time: 30 minutes

Nutritional Value: High in protein, low-carb, and a taste of the Mediterranean.

12. One-Pot Zuppa Toscana

INGREDIENTS

1 lb Italian sausage, crumbled

1 onion, diced

3 cloves garlic, minced

4 cups kale, chopped

4 cups chicken broth

1 cup coconut milk

3 medium potatoes, sliced

Salt and pepper to taste

PREPARATION

In a large pot, brown crumbled Italian sausage over medium heat. Add diced onion and minced garlic. Cook until onion is translucent.

Add chopped kale, chicken broth, coconut milk, and sliced potatoes. Bring to a simmer.

Simmer for 20-25 minutes or until the potatoes are tender.

Season with salt and pepper before serving.

Prep Time: 35 minutes

Nutritional Value: High in protein, low-carb, and a good source of vitamins.

CHAPTER 7: DESSERTS

1. Vanilla-Chamomile Poached Plums

INGREDIENTS

4 plums, halved and pitted

2 cups water

1/2 cup honey or maple syrup

2 chamomile tea bags

1 vanilla bean, split, and seeds scraped

Zest of 1 orange

PREPARATION

In a saucepan, combine water, honey or maple syrup, chamomile tea bags, vanilla bean and seeds, and orange zest.

Bring the mixture to a simmer, stirring until the sweetener is dissolved.

Add plum halves to the simmering liquid. Poach for 5-7 minutes or until plums are tender.

Remove plums and let them cool before serving.

Prep Time: 15 minutes

Nutritional Value: Low-calorie, high in antioxidants, and a good source of vitamins.

2.   Apple-Pear Sauce

INGREDIENTS

4 apples, peeled, cored, and diced

4 pears, peeled, cored, and diced

1/4 cup water

1 teaspoon cinnamon

1/2 teaspoon nutmeg

1 tablespoon honey or maple syrup (optional)

PREPARATION

In a saucepan, combine diced apples, diced pears, water, cinnamon, and nutmeg.

Cook over medium heat until the fruits are soft and easily mashed with a fork.

Mash the fruits to your desired consistency.

If desired, add honey or maple syrup for sweetness.

Allow the sauce to cool before serving.

Prep Time: 20 minutes

Nutritional Value: High in fiber, vitamins, and natural sweetness.

3. Cranberry-Orange Compote

INGREDIENTS

2 cups fresh or frozen cranberries

1/2 cup orange juice

Zest of 1 orange

1/4 cup honey or maple syrup

1 cinnamon stick

PREPARATION

In a saucepan, combine cranberries, orange juice, orange zest, honey or maple syrup, and a cinnamon stick.

Bring the mixture to a simmer over medium heat.

Cook for 10-15 minutes or until the cranberries burst and the compote thickens.

Remove the cinnamon stick and let the compote cool before serving.

Prep Time: 15 minutes

Nutritional Value: High in antioxidants, vitamin C, and natural sweetness.

4. Avocado-Chocolate Frozen Peaches and Cream Bars

INGREDIENTS

2 ripe avocados

1/4 cup cocoa powder

1/4 cup honey or maple syrup

1 teaspoon vanilla extract

1 cup frozen peach slices

PREPARATION

In a blender, combine avocados, cocoa powder, honey or maple syrup, and vanilla extract. Blend until smooth.

In a popsicle mold, layer the avocado-chocolate mixture with frozen peach slices.

Insert popsicle sticks and freeze for at least 4 hours or until solid.

Run the mold under warm water to release the bars before serving.

Prep Time: 15 minutes + freezing time

Nutritional Value: High in healthy fats, antioxidants, and natural sweetness.

5.   Cool Mint and Honeydew Slushy

INGREDIENTS

2 cups honeydew melon, diced

1/2 cup fresh mint leaves

1 tablespoon honey or maple syrup

2 cups ice cubes

1/2 cup cold water

PREPARATION

In a blender, combine honeydew melon, fresh mint leaves, honey or maple syrup, ice cubes, and cold water.

Blend until smooth and slushy.

Pour into glasses and garnish with additional mint leaves if desired.

Serve immediately.

Prep Time: 10 minutes

Nutritional Value: Hydrating, low-calorie, and high in vitamins.

6.   Chocolate-Covered Blueberry-Coconut Bars

INGREDIENTS

1 cup fresh blueberries

1/4 cup shredded coconut

1/4 cup coconut oil, melted

2 tablespoons cocoa powder

1 tablespoon honey or maple syrup

1/2 teaspoon vanilla extract

PREPARATION

Line a small baking dish with parchment paper.

In a bowl, combine fresh blueberries and shredded coconut. Spread evenly in the prepared dish.

In a separate bowl, mix melted coconut oil, cocoa powder, honey or maple syrup, and vanilla extract. Pour over the blueberry-coconut mixture.

Freeze for at least 2 hours or until firm.

Cut into bars and serve.

Prep Time: 15 minutes + freezing time

Nutritional Value: High in antioxidants, healthy fats, and natural sweetness.

7.   Orange Poached Pears with Nutmeg

INGREDIENTS

4 ripe pears, peeled and halved

2 cups orange juice

Zest of 1 orange

1/4 cup honey or maple syrup

1/2 teaspoon ground nutmeg

PREPARATION

In a pot, combine orange juice, orange zest, honey or maple syrup, and ground nutmeg.

Bring the liquid to a simmer over medium heat.

Gently place pear halves in the simmering liquid.

Poach for 15-20 minutes or until the pears are tender.

Remove the pears and let them cool before serving.

Prep Time: 30 minutes

Nutritional Value: High in fiber, vitamin C, and natural sweetness.

CHAPTER 8: KITCHEN STAPLES

1. Coconut Cream

INGREDIENTS

2 cans (14 oz each) full-fat coconut milk

PREPARATION

Chill the cans of coconut milk in the refrigerator overnight.

Open the cans without shaking and scoop out the thick coconut cream that has separated at the top.

Place the coconut cream in a bowl and whip with a hand mixer until smooth.

Use immediately or store in a sealed container in the refrigerator.

Prep Time: 10 minutes (plus chilling time)

Nutritional Value: High in healthy fats and a dairy-free alternative.

2.   Italian Sausage

INGREDIENTS

1 lb ground pork

1 teaspoon fennel seeds

1 teaspoon dried oregano

1 teaspoon dried basil

1/2 teaspoon garlic powder

1/2 teaspoon onion powder

1/2 teaspoon paprika

1/2 teaspoon salt

1/4 teaspoon black pepper

Pinch of red pepper flakes (optional)

PREPARATION

In a bowl, combine ground pork with fennel seeds, dried oregano, dried basil, garlic powder, onion powder, paprika, salt, black pepper, and red pepper flakes if using.

Mix the ingredients well.

Form the mixture into sausage patties or crumbles.

Cook the sausage in a skillet over medium heat until browned and cooked through.

Prep Time: 15 minutes

Nutritional Value: High in protein and free from additives found in commercial sausages.

3. Hard-Boiled Eggs

INGREDIENTS

Eggs

PREPARATION

Place eggs in a single layer in a saucepan or pot.

Cover the eggs with water, ensuring they are fully submerged.

Bring the water to a boil over medium-high heat.

Once boiling, reduce the heat to low and simmer for 10 minutes.

Drain the hot water and transfer the eggs to an ice bath to cool.

Once cooled, peel the eggs.

Prep Time: 15 minutes

Nutritional Value: High in protein, vitamins, and minerals.

4.   Roasted Garlic

INGREDIENTS

Whole garlic bulbs

Olive oil

Salt

PREPARATION

Preheat the oven to 400°F (200°C).

Peel away the loose outer layers of the garlic bulb skin, leaving the skins that are covering the individual cloves.

Cut the top of the garlic bulbs off, exposing the tops of the cloves.

Place the garlic bulbs on a piece of aluminum foil.

Drizzle olive oil over the exposed garlic cloves, letting it soak down into the cloves.

Sprinkle with a pinch of salt.

Wrap the garlic bulbs in the foil and place them in the oven for about 30-40 minutes or until the cloves feel soft when pressed.

Once roasted, let them cool slightly before squeezing out the garlic cloves.

Prep Time: 40 minutes

Nutritional Value: High in antioxidants and adds flavor to dishes.

5.   Slow   Cooker Caramelized Onions

INGREDIENTS

6 large onions, thinly sliced

2 tablespoons olive oil

1/2 teaspoon salt

1/2 teaspoon coconut sugar (optional)

PREPARATION

Place the sliced onions in the slow cooker.

Drizzle olive oil over the onions and sprinkle with salt.

If desired, add coconut sugar for a touch of sweetness.

Stir to coat the onions in oil and seasoning.

Cook on low for 10-12 hours, stirring occasionally, until the onions are golden brown and caramelized.

Prep Time: 10-12 hours (slow cooker time)

Nutritional Value: High in flavor, adds sweetness without added sugars.

6.   Homemade Mayonnaise

INGREDIENTS

1 egg, at room temperature

1 tablespoon Dijon mustard

1 cup light-tasting olive oil or avocado oil

1 tablespoon apple cider vinegar or lemon juice

Salt to taste

PREPARATION

In a blender or food processor, combine the egg and Dijon mustard. Blend until well mixed.

With the blender or food processor running, slowly pour in the oil in a very thin stream until the mixture begins to thicken.

Add apple cider vinegar or lemon juice and continue blending until the mayonnaise reaches the desired consistency.

Season with salt to taste and blend briefly to combine.

Store in a sealed container in the refrigerator.

Prep Time: 10 minutes

Nutritional Value: Homemade mayonnaise is free from artificial additives and can be customized to suit personal taste preferences.

CONCLUSION

The path of a newly diagnosed Hashimoto's thyroiditis can be intimidating, but with the correct understanding and a guided approach, it can become a transformational opportunity.

This book sought to provide a comprehensive knowledge of a Hashimoto's-friendly diet, emphasizing food, balance, and a mindful connection with the body, rather than merely a series of recipes.

Navigating the complexities of Hashimoto's disease entails more than just adjusting to dietary adjustments; it's a journey of self-discovery and empowerment. As we've gone through the dishes, which range from nutrient-dense breakfasts to hearty dinners and delectable sweets, the underlying message has been clear: food can be both medicine and celebration.

We can improve our thyroid health and overall well-being by incorporating nutrient-dense, anti-inflammatory substances. The recipes presented here are more than just instructions; they are an invitation to enjoy the flavors of nourishing, healing foods while cultivating a positive relationship with the act of eating.

Remember that each person's Hashimoto experience is unique, and this guidance serves as a foundation for developing a personalized, long-term approach to a Hashimoto's-friendly diet. Consider this journey to be one of self-care, self-discovery, and a renewed appreciation for the significant impact that mindful eating can have on our health and vitality.

I hope that this book will be a helpful and motivating partner for you as you set out on this life-changing nutritional path. Here's to a life filled with tasty, wholesome choices that encourage you to thrive on Hashimoto's path.

www.ingramcontent.com/pod-product-compliance
Lightning Source LLC
Chambersburg PA
CBHW070943260726
48661CB00003B/1099